Table of Contents

Introduction

My Story

It all started with a dull ache in the chest. I felt like I was walking around with a heavy weight on my shoulders, and I was constantly exhausted. I was too ashamed to tell anyone how I felt, so I chose to ignore it and keep living my life like nothing was wrong.

One day, I heard a friend talking about how diet can affect mental health. I decided to try it out, so I started making small changes to my diet. I cut out processed foods and added more fruits, vegetables, and whole grains. I also made sure to get enough protein and healthy fats.

At first, I didn't feel any different, but slowly I started to feel more energetic and less depressed. I was able to focus better and had more motivation to do things. I even found myself going out more and making more effort to socialize.

I kept up my healthy diet, and before long, my depression was completely gone. I was no longer weighed down by my sadness, and I could feel like myself again. I wasn't sure if it was the diet that helped me, but I'm so grateful that it did.

Now, I make sure to eat a healthy, balanced diet every day. I know that if I ever start to feel down again, I can turn to my diet and give myself the boost I need. It's amazing the power food can have on our mental health, and I'm so glad I learned that lesson.

Everything You Need to Know About Anxiety

Overview

Anxiety is your body's natural response to stress. It's a feeling of fear or apprehension about what's to come. The first day of school, going to a job interview, or giving a speech may cause most people to feel fearful and nervous.

But if your feelings of anxiety are extreme, last for longer than six months, and are interfering with your life, you may have an anxiety disorder.

What are anxiety disorders?

It's normal to feel anxious about moving to a new place, starting a new job, or taking a test. This type of anxiety is unpleasant, but it may motivate you to work harder and to do a better job. Ordinary anxiety is a feeling that comes and goes, but does not interfere with your everyday life.

In the case of an anxiety disorder, the feeling of fear may be with you all the time. It is intense and sometimes debilitating.

This type of anxiety may cause you to stop doing things you enjoy. In extreme cases, it may prevent you from entering an elevator, crossing the street, or even leaving your home. If left untreated, the anxiety will keep getting worse.

Anxiety disorders are the most common form of emotional disorder and can affect anyone at any age. According to the American Psychiatric Association, women are more likely than men to be diagnosed with an anxiety disorder.

What are the types of anxiety disorders?

Anxiety is a key part of several different disorders. These include:

- panic disorder: experiencing recurring panic attacks at unexpected times. A person with panic disorder may live in fear of the next panic attack.

- phobia: excessive fear of a specific object, situation, or activity

- social anxiety disorder: extreme fear of being judged by others in social situations

- obsessive-compulsive disorder: recurring irrational thoughts that lead you to perform specific, repeated behaviors

- separation anxiety disorder: fear of being away from home or loved ones

- illness anxiety disorder: anxiety about your health (formerly called hypochondria)

- post-traumatic stress disorder (PTSD): anxiety following a traumatic event

What are the symptoms of anxiety?

Anxiety feels different depending on the person experiencing it. Feelings can range from butterflies in your stomach to a racing heart. You might feel out of control, like there's a disconnect between your mind and body.

Other ways people experience anxiety include nightmares, panic attacks, and painful thoughts or memories that you can't control. You may have a general feeling of fear and worry, or you may fear a specific place or event.

Symptoms of general anxiety include:

- increased heart rate

- rapid breathing

- restlessness

- trouble concentrating

- difficulty falling asleep

Your anxiety symptoms might be totally different from someone else's. That's why it's important to know all the ways anxiety can present itself.

What is an anxiety attack?

An anxiety attack is a feeling of overwhelming apprehension, worry, distress, or fear. For many people, an anxiety attack builds slowly. It may worsen as a stressful event approaches.

Anxiety attacks can vary greatly, and symptoms may differ among individuals. That's because the many symptoms of anxiety don't happen to everyone, and they can change over time.

Common symptoms of an anxiety attack include:

- feeling faint or dizzy

- shortness of breath

- dry mouth

- sweating

- chills or hot flashes

- apprehension and worry

- restlessness

- distress

- fear

- numbness or tingling

A panic attack and an anxiety attack share some common symptoms, but they're not the same.

What causes anxiety?

Researchers are not sure of the exact cause of anxiety. But, it's likely a combination of factors play a role. These include genetic and environmental factors, as well as brain chemistry.

In addition, researchers believe that the areas of the brain responsible for controlling fear may be impacted.

Current research of anxiety is taking a deeper look at the parts of the brain that are involved with anxiety.

Are there tests that diagnose anxiety?

A single test can't diagnose anxiety. Instead, an anxiety diagnosis requires a lengthy process of physical examinations, mental health evaluations, and psychological questionnaires.

Some doctors may conduct a physical exam, including blood or urine tests to rule out underlying medical conditions that could contribute to symptoms you're experiencing.

Several anxiety tests and scales are also used to help your doctor assess the level of anxiety you're experiencing.

What are treatments for anxiety?

Once you've been diagnosed with anxiety, you can to explore treatment options with your doctor. For some people, medical treatment isn't necessary. Lifestyle changes may be enough to cope with the symptoms.

In moderate or severe cases, however, treatment can help you overcome the symptoms and lead a more manageable day-to-day life.

Treatment for anxiety falls into two categories: psychotherapy and medication. Meeting with a therapist or psychologist can help you learn tools to use and strategies to cope with anxiety when it occurs.

Medications typically used to treat anxiety include antidepressants and sedatives. They work to balance brain chemistry, prevent episodes of anxiety, and ward off the most severe symptoms of the disorder.

What natural remedies are used for anxiety?

Lifestyle changes can be an effective way to relive some of the stress and anxiety you may cope with every day. Most of the natural "remedies" consist of caring for your body, participating in healthy activities, and eliminating unhealthy ones.

These include:

- getting enough sleep

- meditating

- staying active and exercising

- eating a healthy diet

- staying active and working out

- avoiding alcohol

- avoiding caffeine

- quitting smoking cigarettes

If these lifestyle changes seem like a positive way to help you eliminate some anxiety, read about how each one works—

Anxiety and depression

If you have an anxiety disorder, you may also be depressed. While anxiety and depression can occur separately, it's not unusual for these to mental health disorders to happen together.

Anxiety can be a symptom of clinical or major depression. Likewise, worsening symptoms of depression can be triggered by an anxiety disorder.

Symptoms of both conditions can be managed with many of the same treatments: psychotherapy (counseling), medications, and lifestyle changes.

How to help children with anxiety

Anxiety in children is natural and common. In fact, one in eight children will experience anxiety. As children grow up and learn from their parents, friends, and caretakers, they typically develop the skills to calm themselves and cope with feelings of anxiety.

But, anxiety in children can also become chronic and persistent, developing into an anxiety disorder. Uncontrolled anxiety may begin to interfere with daily activities, and children may avoid interacting with their peers or family members.

Symptoms of an anxiety disorder might include:

- jitteriness

- irritability

- sleeplessness

- feelings of fear

- shame

- feelings of isolation

Anxiety treatment for children includes cognitive behavioral therapy (talk therapy) and medications.

How to help teens with anxiety

Teenagers may have many reasons to be anxious. Tests, college visits, and first dates all pop up in these important years. But teenagers who feel anxious or experience symptoms of anxiety frequently may have an anxiety disorder.

Symptoms of anxiety in teenagers may include nervousness, shyness, isolationist behaviors, and avoidance. Likewise, anxiety in teens may lead to unusual behaviors. They may act out, perform poorly in school, skip social events, and even engage in substance or alcohol use.

For some teens, depression may accompany anxiety. Diagnosing both conditions is important so that treatment can address the underlying issues and help relieve symptoms.

The most common treatments for anxiety in teenagers are talk therapy and medication. These treatments also help address depression symptoms.

Anxiety and stress

Stress and anxiety are two sides of the same coin. Stress is the result of demands on your brain or body. It can be the caused by an event or activity that makes you nervous or worrisome. Anxiety is that same worry, fear, or unease.

Anxiety can be a reaction to your stress, but it can also occur in people who have no obvious stressors.

Both anxiety and stress cause physical and mental symptoms. These include:

- headache

- stomachache

- fast heartbeat

- sweating

- dizziness

- jitteriness

- muscle tension

- rapid breathing

- panic

- nervousness

- difficulty concentrating

- irrational anger or irritability

- restlessness

- sleeplessness

Neither stress nor anxiety is always bad. Both can actually provide you with a bit of a boost or incentive to accomplish the task or challenge before you. However, if they become persistent, they can begin to interfere with your daily life. In that case, it's important to seek treatment.

The long-term outlook for untreated depression and anxiety includes chronic health issues, such as heart disease.

Anxiety and alcohol

If you're anxious frequently, you may decide you'd like a drink to calm your nerves. After all, alcohol is a sedative. It can depress the activity of your central nervous system, which may help you feel more relaxed.

In a social setting, that may feel like just the answer you need to let down your guard. Ultimately, it may not be the best solution.

Some people with anxiety disorders end up abusing alcohol or other drugs in an effort to feel better regularly. This can create a dependency and addiction.

It may be necessary to treat an alcohol or drug problem before the anxiety can be addressed. Chronic or long-term use can ultimately make the condition worse, too.

Can foods treat anxiety?

Medication and talk therapy are commonly used to treat anxiety. Lifestyle changes, like getting enough sleep and regular exercise, can also help. In addition, some research suggests the foods you eat may have a beneficial impact on your brain if you frequently experience anxiety.

These foods include:

- salmon

- chamomile

- turmeric

- dark chocolate

- yogurt

- green tea

Outlook

Anxiety disorders can be treated with medication, psychotherapy, or a combination of the two. Some people who have a mild anxiety disorder, or a fear of something they can easily avoid, decide to live with the condition and to not seek treatment.

It's important to understand that anxiety disorders can be treated, even in severe cases. Although, anxiety usually doesn't go away, you can learn to manage it and live a happy, healthy life.

6 Foods That Help Reduce Anxiety

Anxiety is a common problem for many people.

It's a disorder characterized by constant worry and nervousness, and is sometimes related to poor brain health. Medication is often required as treatment.

Aside from medication, there are several strategies you can use to help reduce anxiety symptoms, from exercising to deep breathing.

Additionally, there are some foods you can eat that may help lower the severity of your symptoms, mostly due to their brain-boosting properties.

Here are 6 science-backed foods and beverages that may provide anxiety relief.

1. Salmon

Salmon may be beneficial for reducing anxiety.

It contains nutrients that promote brain health, including vitamin D and the omega-3 fatty acids eicosapentaenoic acid (EPA) and docosahexaenoic acid (DHA).

EPA and DHA may help regulate the neurotransmitters dopamine and serotonin, which can have calming and relaxing properties.

Additionally, studies show these fatty acids can reduce inflammation and prevent brain cell dysfunction that leads to the development of mental disorders like anxiety.

Consuming adequate amounts of EPA and DHA may also promote your brain's ability to adapt to changes, allowing you to better handle stressors that trigger anxiety symptoms.

Vitamin D has also been studied for the positive effects it may have on improving levels of calming neurotransmitters.

Even a few servings of salmon a week may be enough to promote anxiety relief.

In one study, men who ate Atlantic salmon three times per week for five months reported less anxiety than those who ate chicken, pork or beef. Moreover, they had improved anxiety-related symptoms, such as heart rate and heart rate variability.

SUMMARY:

Salmon is high in omega-3 fatty acids and vitamin D, which may assist in anxiety relief by promoting brain health.

2. Chamomile

Chamomile is an herb that may help reduce anxiety.

It contains high amounts of antioxidants proven to reduce inflammation, which might decrease the risk of anxiety.

Several studies have examined the association between chamomile and anxiety relief.

They've found that those diagnosed with generalized anxiety disorder (GAD) experienced a significantly greater reduction in symptoms after consuming chamomile extract, compared to those who did not.

Another study found similar results, as those who consumed chamomile extract for eight weeks saw reduced symptoms of depression and anxiety.

While these results are promising, most studies have been conducted on chamomile extract. More research is necessary to evaluate the anti-anxiety effects of chamomile tea, which is most commonly consumed.

SUMMARY:

Chamomile has been shown to help with anxiety reduction due to its antioxidant content and anti-inflammatory effects.

3. Turmeric

Turmeric is a spice that contains curcumin, a compound studied for its role in promoting brain health and preventing anxiety disorders.

Animal and test-tube studies suggest that curcumin may boost the omega-3 fatty acid DHA in the brain by helping your body synthesize it more efficiently.

In one study, 20 mg/kg of curcumin produced significant anti-anxiety effects in stressed mice compared to those given a lower dose.

Curcumin also has powerful antioxidant and anti-inflammatory properties that have been shown to prevent damage to brain cells.

These effects are partly due to curcumin's ability to reduce inflammatory markers, such as cytokines, which are often linked with anxiety development

Additionally, curcumin consumption has been shown to increase blood antioxidant levels, which tend to be low in individuals with anxiety.

More human research is needed to confirm all of these effects, but if you suffer from anxiety, incorporating turmeric into your diet is certainly worth a try.

SUMMARY:

Turmeric contains curcumin, a compound with antioxidant and anti-inflammatory properties that may alleviate anxiety symptoms.

4. Dark Chocolate

Incorporating some dark chocolate into your diet may also be helpful for easing anxiety.

Dark chocolate contains flavonols, which are antioxidants that may benefit brain function.

They do this by improving blood flow to the brain and promoting its ability to adapt to stressful situations.

These effects may allow you to adjust better to the stressful situations that can lead to anxiety and other mood disorders.

Some researchers also suggest that dark chocolate's role in brain health may simply be due to its taste, which can be comforting for those with mood disorders.

In one study, individuals who consumed 74% dark chocolate twice daily for two weeks had improved levels of stress hormones commonly associated with anxiety, such as catecholamines and cortisol.

Eating dark chocolate has also been shown to increase levels of the neurotransmitter serotonin, which may help reduce the stress that leads to anxiety.

For example, in a study of highly stressed individuals, participants reported significantly lower levels of stress after consuming 40 grams of dark chocolate every day over a two-week period.

However, dark chocolate is best consumed in moderation, as it is high in calories and easy to overeat. 1–1.5 ounces is a reasonable serving size.

SUMMARY:

Dark chocolate may be helpful for improving anxiety due to its stress-reducing antioxidants and ability to increase serotonin levels.

5. Yogurt

If you suffer from anxiety, yogurt is a great food to include in your diet.

The probiotics, or healthy bacteria, found in some types of yogurt can improve several aspects of your well-being, including mental health.

Studies have shown that probiotic foods like yogurt may promote mental health and brain function by inhibiting free radicals and neurotoxins, which can damage nerve tissue in the brain and lead to anxiety.

In one study, anxious individuals who consumed probiotic yogurt daily were better able to cope with stress than those who consumed yogurt without probiotics.

Another study found that women who consumed 4.4 ounces (125 grams) of yogurt twice daily for four weeks had better functioning of the brain regions that control emotion and sensation, which may be associated with lower anxiety levels.

These findings are promising, but more human research is necessary to confirm the beneficial effects that yogurt may have on anxiety reduction.

It is also important to note that not all yogurt contains probiotics. For the benefits of probiotics, choose a yogurt that has live active cultures listed as an ingredient.

SUMMARY: Yogurt contains probiotics, which may have a positive effect on brain health and anxiety levels.

6. Green Tea

Green tea contains L-theanine, an amino acid that has been studied for the positive effects it may have on brain health and anxiety reduction.

In one small study, people who consumed L-theanine experienced a reduction in psychological stress responses that are commonly associated with anxiety, such as increased heart rate.

Another study found that those who drank a beverage that contained L-theanine had decreased levels of cortisol, a stress hormone linked with anxiety.

These effects may be due to L-theanine's potential to prevent nerves from becoming overexcited. Additionally, L-theanine may increase GABA, dopamine and serotonin, neurotransmitters that have been shown to have anti-anxiety effects.

Moreover, green tea contains epigallocatechin gallate (EGCG), an antioxidant suggested to promote brain health. It may play a role in reducing certain symptoms by also increasing GABA in the brain.

One mouse study found that EGCG produced anti-anxiety effects similar to those of common anxiety medications.

The beneficial properties of L-theanine and EGCG may be a major reason why drinking several cups of green tea daily is associated with less psychological distress.

While all of these findings are promising, it is worth mentioning that most of the research on green tea and anxiety has been conducted in animals and test tubes. More human research is needed to confirm its anti-anxiety effects.

SUMMARY:Green tea contains L-theanine and EGCG, which may promote brain health and anxiety reduction.

Other Foods That May Help With Anxiety

While some of the foods listed below have not been studied specifically for their anti-anxiety effects, they are rich in nutrients thought to improve related symptoms.

• Turkey, bananas and oats: These are good sources of the amino acid tryptophan, which is converted to serotonin in the body and may promote relaxation and anxiety relief.

• Eggs, meat and dairy products: All provide high-quality protein including essential amino acids that produce the neurotransmitters dopamine and serotonin, which have the potential to improve mental health .

• Chia seeds: Chia seeds are another good source of brain-boosting omega-

3 fatty acids, which have been shown to help with anxiety.

• Citrus fruits and bell peppers: These fruits are rich in vitamin C, which has antioxidant properties that may help reduce inflammation and prevent damage to cells that may promote anxiety.

• Almonds: Almonds provide a significant amount of vitamin E, which has been studied for its role in anxiety prevention.

• Blueberries: Blueberries are high in vitamin C and other antioxidants, such as flavonoids, that have been studied for their ability to improve brain health and thus help with anxiety relief.

SUMMARY: Some foods contain specific nutrients that may promote brain health and help prevent anxiety or reduce the severity of your symptoms.

The Bottom Line

Overall, research is sparse on the topic of specific foods and anxiety prevention.

Most studies have been conducted on animals or in laboratories, and more high-quality human studies are needed.

However, there are several foods and beverages that may help you deal with your anxiety symptoms, as they may reduce inflammation and boost brain health.

18 Terrific Foods to Help Relieve Stress

If you're feeling stressed, it's only natural to seek relief.

While occasional bouts of stress are difficult to avoid, chronic stress can take a serious toll on your physical and emotional health. In fact, it may increase your risk of conditions like heart disease and depression.

Interestingly, certain foods and beverages may have stress-relieving qualities.

Here are 18 stress-relieving foods and beverages to add to your diet.

1. Matcha powder

This vibrant green tea powder is popular among health enthusiasts because it's rich in L-theanine, a non-protein amino acid with powerful stress-relieving properties.

Matcha is a better source of this amino acid than other types of green tea, as it's made from green tea leaves grown in shade. This process increases its content of certain compounds, including L-theanine.

Both human and animal studies show that matcha may reduce stress if its L-theanine content is high enough and its caffeine is low.

For example, in a 15-day study, 36 people ate cookies containing 4.5 grams of matcha powder each day. They experienced significantly reduced activity of the stress marker salivary alpha-amylase, compared with a placebo group.

2. Swiss chard

Swiss chard is a leafy green vegetable that's packed with stress-fighting nutrients.

Just 1 cup (175 grams) of cooked Swiss chard contains 36% of the recommended intake for magnesium, which plays an important role in your body's stress response.

Low levels of this mineral are associated with conditions like anxiety and panic attacks. Plus, chronic stress may deplete your body's magnesium stores, making this mineral especially important when you're stressed.

3. Sweet potatoes

Eating whole, nutrient-rich carb sources like sweet potatoes may help lower levels of the stress hormone cortisol.

Although cortisol levels are tightly regulated, chronic stress can lead to cortisol dysfunction, which may cause inflammation, pain, and other adverse effects.

An 8-week study in women with excess weight or obesity found that those who ate a diet rich in whole, nutrient-dense carbs had significantly lower levels of salivary cortisol than those who followed a standard American diet high in refined carbs.

Sweet potatoes are a whole food that makes an excellent carb choice. They're packed with nutrients that are important for stress response, such as vitamin C and potassium.

4. Kimchi

Kimchi is a fermented vegetable dish that's typically made with napa cabbage and daikon, a type of radish. Fermented foods like kimchi are packed with beneficial bacteria called probiotics and high in vitamins, minerals, and antioxidants.

Research reveals that fermented foods may help reduce stress and anxiety. For example, in a study in 710 young adults, those who ate fermented foods more frequently experienced fewer symptoms of social anxiety.

Many other studies show that probiotic supplements and probiotic-rich foods like kimchi have beneficial effects on mental health. This is likely due to their interactions with your gut bacteria, which directly affect your mood.

5. Artichokes

Artichokes are an incredibly concentrated source of fiber and especially rich in prebiotics, a type of fiber that feeds the friendly bacteria in your gut.

Animal studies indicate that prebiotics like fructooligosaccharides (FOSs), which are concentrated in artichokes, may help reduce stress levels.

Plus, one review demonstrated that people who ate 5 or more grams of prebiotics per day experienced improved anxiety and depression symptoms, as well as that high quality, prebiotic-rich diets may reduce your risk of stress.

Artichokes are also high in potassium, magnesium, and vitamins C and K, all of which are essential for a healthy stress response.

6. Organ meats

Organ meats, which include the heart, liver, and kidneys of animals like cows and chickens, are an excellent source of B vitamins, especially B12, B6, riboflavin, and folate, which are essential for stress control.

For example, B vitamins are necessary for the production of neurotransmitters like dopamine and serotonin, which help regulate mood.

Supplementing with B vitamins or eating foods like organ meats may help reduce stress. A review of 18 studies in adults found that B vitamin supplements lowered stress levels and significantly benefited mood.

Just 1 slice (85 grams) of beef liver delivers over 50% of the Daily Value (DV) for vitamin B6 and folate, over

200% of the DV for riboflavin, and over 2,000% of the DV for vitamin B12.

7. Eggs

Eggs are often referred to as nature's multivitamin because of their impressive nutrient profile. Whole eggs are packed with vitamins, minerals, amino acids, and antioxidants needed for a healthy stress response.

Whole eggs are particularly rich in choline, a nutrient found in large amounts in only a few foods. Choline has been shown to play an important role in brain health and may protect against stress.

Animal studies note that choline supplements may aid stress response and boost mood (25Trusted Source).

8. Shellfish

Shellfish, which include mussels, clams, and oysters, are high in amino acids like taurine, which has been studied for its potential mood-boosting properties.

Taurine and other amino acids are needed to produce neurotransmitters like dopamine, which are essential for regulating stress response. In fact, studies indicate that taurine may have antidepressant effects.

Shellfish are also loaded with vitamin B12, zinc, copper, manganese, and selenium, all of which may help boost mood. A study in 2,089 Japanese adults associated low intakes of zinc, copper, and manganese with depression and anxiety symptoms.

9. Acerola cherry powder

Acerola cherries are one of the most concentrated sources of vitamin C.

They boast 50–100% more vitamin C than citrus fruits like oranges and lemons (.

Vitamin C is involved in stress response. What's more, high vitamin C levels are linked to elevated mood and lower levels of depression and anger. Plus, eating foods rich in this vitamin may improve overall mood.

Although they can be enjoyed fresh, acerola cherries are highly perishable. As such, they're most often sold as a powder, which you can add to foods and beverages.

10. Fatty fish

Fatty fish like mackerel, herring, salmon, and sardines are incredibly rich in omega-3 fats and vitamin D, nutrients that have been shown to help reduce stress levels and improve mood.

Omega-3s are not only essential for brain health and mood but may also help your body handle stress. In fact, low omega-3 intake is linked to increased anxiety and depression in Western populations.

Vitamin D also plays critical roles in mental health and stress regulation. Low levels are associated with an increased risk of anxiety and depression.

11. Parsley

Parsley is a nutritious herb that's packed with antioxidants — compounds that neutralize unstable molecules called free radicals and protect against oxidative stress.

Oxidative stress is associated with many illnesses, including mental health disorders like depression and anxiety. Studies suggest that a diet rich in antioxidants may help prevent stress and anxiety.

Antioxidants can also help reduce inflammation, which is often high in those with chronic stress.

Parsley is especially rich in carotenoids, flavonoids, and volatile oils, all of which have powerful antioxidant properties.

12. Garlic

Garlic is high in sulfur compounds that help increase levels of glutathione.

This antioxidant is part of your body's first line of defense against stress.

What's more, animal studies suggest that garlic helps combat stress and reduce symptoms of anxiety and depression. Still, more human research is needed.

How to Peel Garlic

13. Tahini

Tahini is a rich spread made from sesame seeds, which are an excellent source of the amino acid L-tryptophan.

L-tryptophan is a precursor of the mood-regulating neurotransmitters dopamine and serotonin. Following a diet high in tryptophan may help boost mood and ease symptoms of depression and anxiety.

In a 4-day study in 25 young adults, a high tryptophan diet led to better mood, decreased anxiety, and reduced depression symptoms, compared with a diet low in this amino acid.

14. Sunflower seeds

Sunflower seeds are a rich source of vitamin E. This fat-soluble vitamin acts as a powerful antioxidant and is essential for mental health.

A low intake of this nutrient is associated with altered mood and depression.

Sunflower seeds are also high in other stress-reducing nutrients, including magnesium, manganese, selenium, zinc, B vitamins, and copper.

15. Broccoli

Cruciferous vegetables like broccoli are renowned for their health benefits.

A diet rich in cruciferous vegetables

may lower your risk of certain cancers, heart disease, and mental health disorders like depression.

Cruciferous vegetables like broccoli are some of the most concentrated food sources of some nutrients — including magnesium, vitamin C, and folate — that have been proven to combat depressive symptoms.

Broccoli is also rich in sulforaphane, a sulfur compound that has neuroprotective properties and may offer calming and antidepressant effects.

Additionally, 1 cup (184 grams) of cooked broccoli packs over 20% of the DV for vitamin B6, a higher intake of which is tied to a lower risk of anxiety and depression in women.

16. Chickpeas

Chickpeas are packed with stress-fighting vitamins and minerals, including magnesium, potassium, B vitamins, zinc, selenium, manganese, and copper.

These delicious legumes are also rich in L-tryptophan, which your body needs to produce mood-regulating neurotransmitters.

Research has found that diets rich in plant proteins like chickpeas may help boost brain health and improve mental performance.

In a study in over 9,000 people, those who followed a Mediterranean diet rich in plant foods like legumes experienced better mood and less stress than those who followed a typical Western diet rich in processed foods.

17. Chamomile tea

Chamomile is a medicinal herb that has been used since ancient times as a natural stress reducer. Its tea and extract have been shown to promote restful sleep and reduce symptoms of anxiety and depression.

An 8-week study in 45 people with anxiety demonstrated that taking 1.5 grams of chamomile extract reduced salivary cortisol levels and improved anxiety symptoms.

18. Blueberries

Blueberries are associated with a number of health benefits, including improved mood.

These berries are high in flavonoid antioxidants that have powerful anti-inflammatory and neuroprotective effects. They may help reduce stress-related inflammation and protect against stress-related cellular damage.

What's more, studies have shown that eating flavonoid-rich foods like blueberries may safeguard against depression and boost your mood.

The bottom line

Numerous foods contain nutrients that may help you reduce stress.

Matcha powder, fatty fish, kimchi, garlic, chamomile tea, and broccoli are just a few that may help.

Try incorporating some of these foods and beverages into your diet to naturally promote stress relief.

www.ingramcontent.com/pod-product-compliance
Lightning Source LLC
Chambersburg PA
CBHW071023260726
48662CB00024B/1788